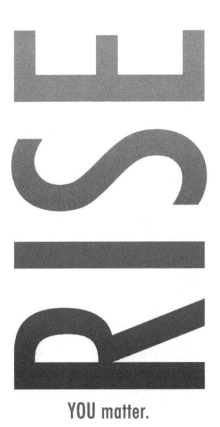

YOU matter.

Candice Nicole

RISE, You Matter
RISE, you matter

About the Author

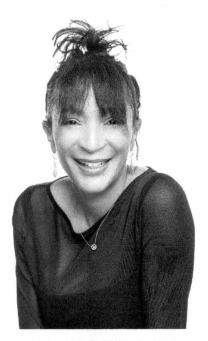

Candice Nicole has been health-focused from early childhood, from foods to fitness. She became a veteran of the health, wellness, and fitness industry; and is Founder and President of a plant-based mineral nutrition company with domestic and international outlets focused on whole-life wellness.

Prior to health and wellness, Candice had careers in technology, marketing and real estate as an investor and developer. It is her belief that when we are helping others, genuinely and sincerely, we are experiencing our greatest joy.

RISE was divinely inspired and born out of a monthly healthy choice newsletter and copious notes taken over time from the road, in airports, hotel rooms, trains, eatery windows, and some restless homebound evenings. RISE is a table-in-waiting, positive-purposed read for every family room, spa hang, poolside pleasure, practitioner cool time, last leg flight, or anytime a personal positive is requisite.

With a goal of living our optimal lives, filled with what most will call

RISE, you matter

happiness—and what Candice terms as JOY—which leads to many positive outcomes, for you and all in your paths. RISE intends to take the reader on an internal in-depth personal thought provoking discovery of self. Tapping into and exploring how we can increase our joy and journeys. How we treat ourselves, how we treat others, how we allow others to affect our treatment of ourselves, and how each individual's actions, words, and even expressions determine destinies that lift or lower.

Candice's mission is to live a healthy, purpose-filled life. Giving birth to RISE Corporation is continuing the journey and its mission is similar. To assist others in living more purpose-filled lives by delivering RISE and other books, cards, stationery, and paper goods with a focus on fun, positive words and messages that lend and lead to renewed thoughts, that evoke and provoke changed hearts and benevolent behavior for all RISE readers.

Whether tears of troubled times or hilltop highlights, rising behavior can lead to outcomes that decidedly and positively shape individuals, relationships, households, workplaces, social media threads – the world.

Each person has the power to affect great change. It starts with sincere, kind, genuine thought and requires heart, sometimes words (because words can be taciturn) and actions.

Words matter. Actions matter. YOU matter.

You decide what positive difference(s) you will make – that will make YOUR journey matter the most.

RISE.

Note from the Author

Thank you for selecting RISE for your table or a gift.

We are all on different paths. Where ever you may be on your journey, as you turn the pages of RISE may the words you read here inspire your personal best. Perhaps propel new horizons.

My intention - to create a timeless gift, for self or another. A beneficial powerfully packed, coffee table read, where thought is induced on each page, at every read, no matter the readers current station. A book that produces real time initial and abiding thought, offering lifetime nuggets of wisdom you can refer back to time and time again.

My hope - RISE provides positivity and purpose in life-altering ways that increase love at large, self-love, growth, forgiveness, mindfulness and reflection, daily or often. It is important to know who you are, to have joy in life, to know you are valuable, to genuinely give back and paramount, to find and live into your purpose.

Memorizing pages that speak to you may provide new ways of thinking and living. Personally, to aid memory, I have found mnemonic devices beneficial. I have inserted "notes" pages along the way for note takers who may find inscription helpful for jotting reminders or "to do's" that resonate.

Get ready to RISE.

RISE, you matter

RISE, you matter

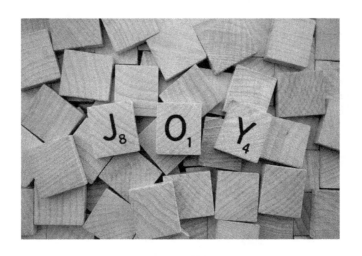

EVERY   SINGLE   DAY.

RISE, you matter

RISE, you matter

Forward

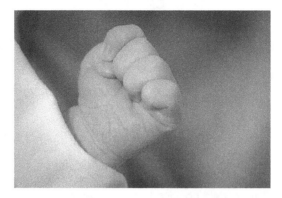

We come in with tight little fist, we leave with hands wide open.

Along the journey, we will laugh and cry, love and lose, dream and discover, romp around and work hard at times.

What will matter most is the JOY we will allow ourselves to live in so that we can live, lead and leave memories that are thought about, spoken of and recalled often with delectation.

What does your JOY life look like?

Are you living in JOY every single day?

RISE, you matter

DEDICATION

Mom,

In youth there is a lack of knowing. I came to know your incredible strength and your sound reasoning. Thank you for the shelter, for teaching me there is something bigger and for planting in me strong necessary roots, even against my will at times, that would ultimately enable me to muster that strength to navigate my life's joyful purposes.

May I continue to yield positive harvest, every day.

ANK,

Thank you for growing me. You have made me a stronger human being and taught me what real and unconditional love truly is. I love you now, always and forever, no matter where you go or what you do. You are my greatest gift. Forever.

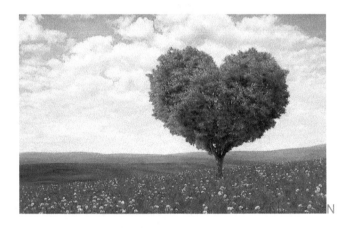

RISE, you matter

ACKNOWLEDGMENTS

Thank you,

Bryon Gold, Paul Grady, Roland Gustavsson, Debbie and Richard Lanich-Labrea, ZV. Lipman, Linda Lull, Dr. Ana Marx, Michael Paparella, Dr. Susan Salem, Sandy Sykes, Chris Wzaczack ...

... when I did not always know the how, the why, the when, the where, the what, and the who .... your genuine, kind, selfless support meant and means more than words will ever articulate. I see your beauty, grace and light. I love you.

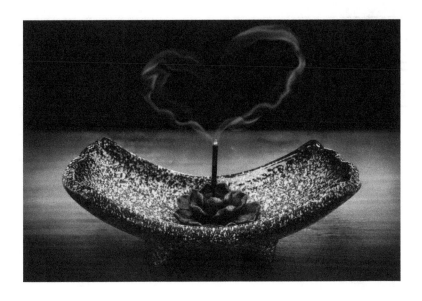

RISE, you matter

Thoughts to note …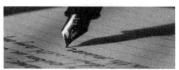

———————————————————————————
———————————————————————————
———————————————————————————
———————————————————————————
———————————————————————————
———————————————————————————
———————————————————————————
———————————————————————————
———————————————————————————
———————————————————————————
———————————————————————————

Opening

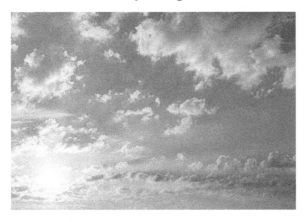

Look up, look up

you miss so much ….

Put the "to do's" and the phone down

see and be seen …

Turn everything around.

Walk with your head held high - gaze straight

Your destiny will not be late!

C. Nicole

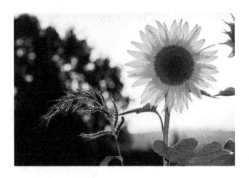

Hopelessness causes great and grave circumstances.

This is why LOVE and KINDNESS are so salient and should be the law of the land – again.

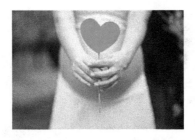

Messages are imprinted on us in our infancy. If we are not cognizant we spend our entire life – wasting moments of joy – trying to decipher, justify, lay culpability and eradicate the imperfect, that does have its purpose.

There is no perfect, just lessons to get us to and through our mission successfully. Answers won't come until we are living in the present. They will come quicker if we are living in the present, in joy. Then, seemingly out of nowhere we will have "moments of clarifying understanding" answering all our "why is this or did these" moments or memories have its time with us.

Do not let those "why" moments and memories stain you or have more time with you than necessary. It stops your progress and is a time waster you can never get back.

The freedom is in the decision to live in the joy moment and not past pains that we either had no choice in or could not understand how best to manage at our infancy – whatever that age or stage.

As wisdom is gained, we get to make better choices that can change our stories monumentally.

If you are anywhere other than on the path of doing the work that allows you to live in joy and purpose, right now – REVERSE DIRECTION.

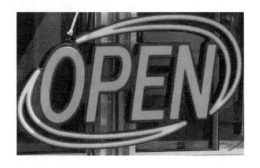

Make yourself available and vulnerable.

Watch the soul grow.

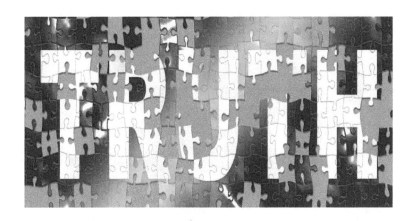

A soul invaded with the truth is truly free.

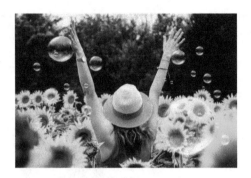

Happiness really means JOY.

True JOY comes from values instilled and the soul. It shines through your spirit and it can not be contained.

You can have JOY every single day - no matter what. It is a decision you make.

JOY can be seen in the eye, in speech, in your walk and how you show up in life. It radiates externally, like a beam of light.

Be luminescent.

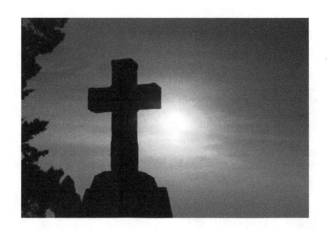

Spirit - the intellect of the soul.

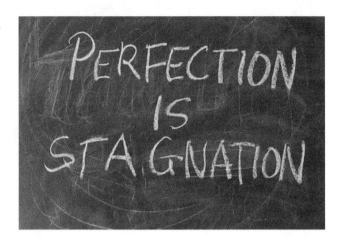

Thank goodness you are not your pant size, bank account, the house you reside in, the car you drive, the length of your hair, the shape of your nose, your skin color, your athletic ability, your vocabulary or the language you speak - you are SO MUCH MORE.

It is your HEART, your SOUL and most important, your SPIRIT that leads your intention and propels your works – that's what makes you, YOU.

Make a note!

Thoughts to note ...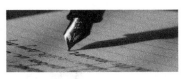

_____

_____

_____

_____

_____

_____

_____

_____

_____

_____

_____

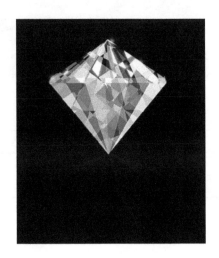

We are all flawed - because we are HUman.

So what, keep growing.

Remember to love and be KIND along the way.

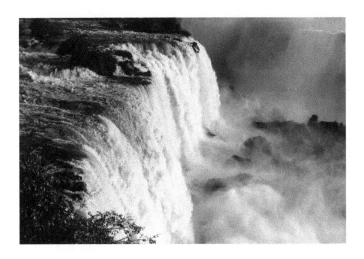

To all things do not do the least, whether a workout, homework or an unexpected call of duty - to these and all things, excel and exceed.

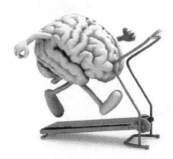

Wholeness – You progress in life by learning and movement.

We work on the outward physical appearance, often disregarding the inward.

The **physical**, **mental** and **spiritual** must align. Building the outward temple is important. However, it will not hold its merits without the inward work.

Important to run and read!

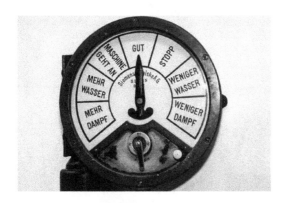

It is wise to remember, you cannot command your feelings.

You can only command your will.

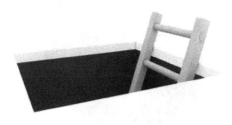

What makes you smile inside, with zero effort?

That's what 90% of your day and life should look and feel like.

Climb up and out - take the position in life you were born to possess.

Hold your head high.

Up, up to the sky.

Be observant ...... for observation breeds inspiration.

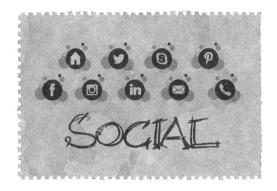

It does not matter if millions or billions LIKE and FOLLOW you. At some point YOU will have to make the conscious decision to do what YOUR internal, intellectual common sense radar says is correct and right for YOU - emotionally, ethically, financially, morally and spiritually.

It is not wise to conform to the possibly diluted, distorted, dysfunctional dire in the world. It may have no or miniscule contribution to your outcome, unless of course, you choose otherwise.

Live life in your lane and on your terms. Do not be consumed with the inconsequential "likes' and "followers". It will create road blocks that amount to loneliness, lacking and perpetual circling.

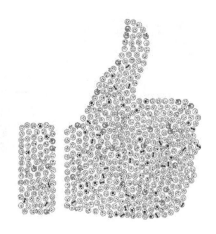

To say I can, is determination in the heart and mind.

Even when you don't know the how, the when, the why, the where, or the what …. it is determination in the heart and mind that stays the course.

If you believe you can't, you won't.

If you believe you can, you will.

Stay determined and effect oriented.

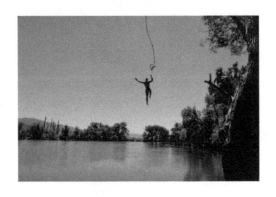

Without progress and growth it is hard to have JOY.

Thoughts to note ...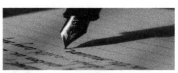

_____

_____

_____

_____

_____

_____

_____

_____

_____

_____

_____

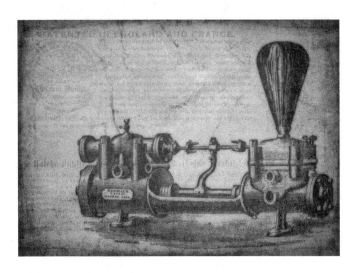

Some things are knowable - pay attention.

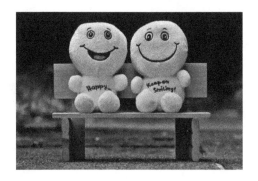

Everyone, at some point, is experiencing challenge.

Daily, walk in life with an internal smile, no matter what.

NO

MATTER

WHAT!!!

It will be apparent in your face and it will change every circumstance - for you and for others.

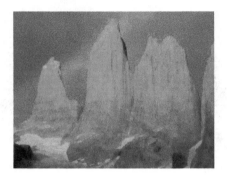

Sometimes pain has a smile, says everything is well, and outwardly does the daily with expected familiarity.

Pain won't ever be agreeable, for it is temporarily disconnected.

Observe and listen with your soul.

Lenient **persistence, kindness, connection** and a **judge free** heart are requisite.

The soul will tell you when everything is well.

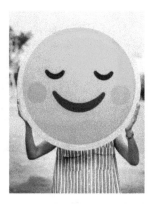

When your spirit is smiling, it shows on your face, even when there is no physical outward apparent smile.

SMILE, at 5 AM as you must start your day.

SMILE when you enter the elevator and blank, unapproachable faces stare back … say hello.

SMILE when checking out at the supermarket and you realize you forgot your wallet, SMILE and be patient if you are the next in line.

SMILE when you realize coffee stains adorn your garment as you enter the important meeting.

SMILE at the end of the long bike ride and it's all uphill.

SMILE when the mechanic gives you the news, and get a second opinion.

SMILE and remember, it will make every circumstance better.

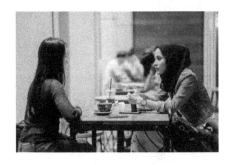

Don't downplay, dodge, be distant or deminimis when someone is sharing with you how THEY feel.

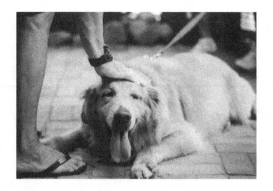

You don't have to be brilliant, beautiful, wealthy, or perfect to help someone. YOU just have to care.

Care, Caring = compassion and humility.

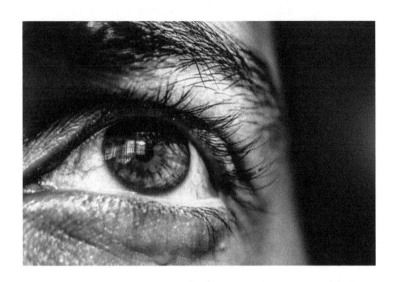

It is OK and possible to be angry and KIND - at the same time.

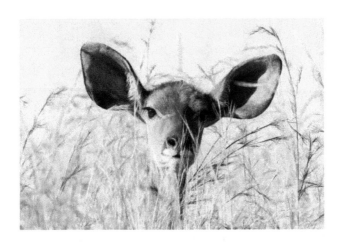

Listen

There is a reason we have two ears.

Lean in - *and* really listen.

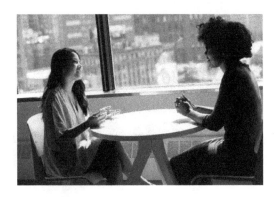

When another has the floor do not overshadow their share time. It is their important story and their time.

Set aside competitive disruptive interjections and the need to share your "similar", "better" or off topic highlights.

It is rude and it is not your time.

Wait your turn, and more importantly, the proper timing.

Even if it is another day.

Thoughts to note ...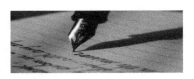

_____

_____

_____

_____

_____

_____

_____

_____

_____

_____

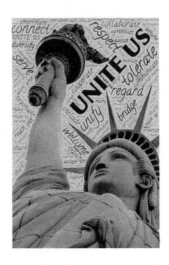

Nothing good can come and remain if you do not have respect and transparency.

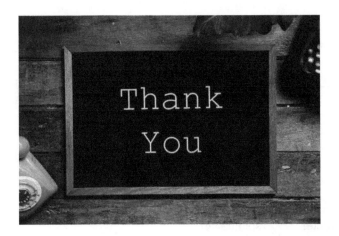

Just say THANK YOU – when someone makes an inappropriate statement or ask a personal or inappropriate question ...... and SMILE.

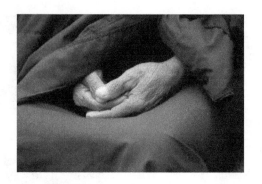

Character   (spirituality)

Experience   (education)

Timing   (preparation)

→   Destiny

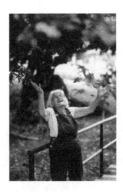

What is happy?

A momentary or situational feeling when a day has gone well, you receive a gift, get the job, get the deal, win the game, the girl, the boy or the prize.

When you live in each moment, hour, day, week, month and year and the **right now** - you learn, you grow, develop grace and come to understand sometimes words and things are not required. It is being content in that moment right then – as it is happening, taking it in.

This is the *real win*.

It produces and is JOY, which is the real producer of feeling "happy".

Happiness usually comes in suddenly. It is momentary to short prolonged situational periods and it is transitory.

Joy is every single day, all day, in any situation.

Seek JOY.

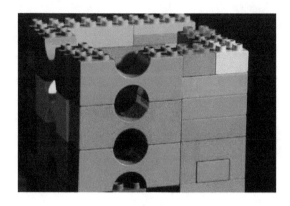

Some of our favorite childhood toys were ones that caused the most grievance. The challenge of the square and round holes game with the odd shaped pegs to strategically fit. Our awkward tiny hands and limited coping measures. Ah, what fun!

Something to commemorate: If our plans do not always align with our better than best efforts, best not to forcefully challenge.

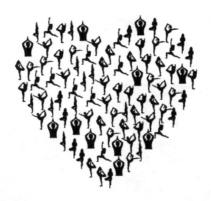

Stretch yourself farther than you think you can.

Then stretch some more.

And some more.

Replicate daily.

Body I Mind I Spirit

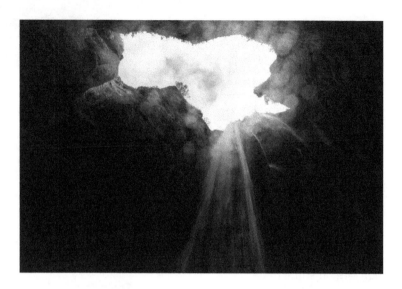

There is untapped space deep inside you. Waiting to be unleashed.

Be present, be quiet and be conscious. Look, listen, learn and let growth and knowledge lead you to your soul, which will lead you to your purpose. You will feel it happening.

Growth and knowledge will come in different forms. Sometimes in other souls to help YOU tap into YOU.

Be mindful.

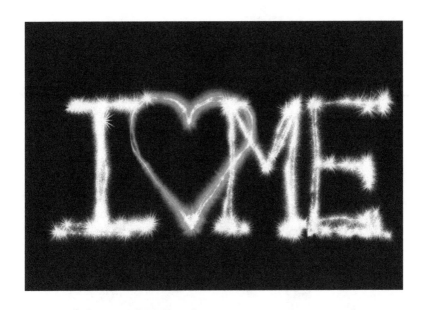

Self, can be the most troubled weed in the garden.

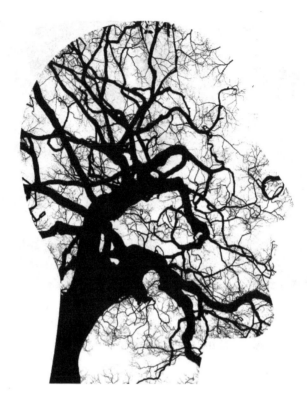

Wise counsel aids recovery.

Thoughts to note …

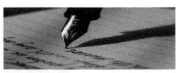

_____

_____

_____

_____

_____

_____

_____

_____

_____

_____

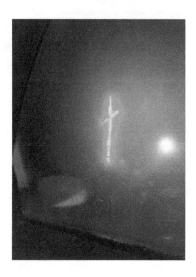

The human condition can weather any storm, with prayer and meditation.

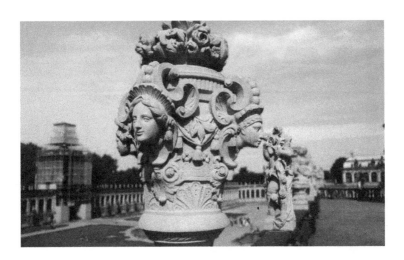

Truth + Time = Love and Restoration.

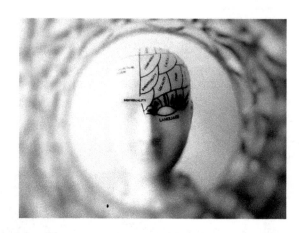

Grow your mind, grow your body - you grow your life.

Transformation of the mind is a MUST!

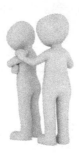

A stubborn mindset is a great enemy of peace

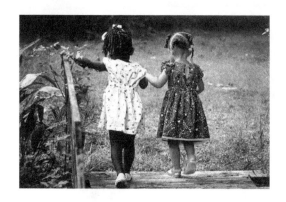

There is a difference between childish and child-like.

Like a child, always be agog and maintain a childlike heart and spirit …

open,

innocent,

loving,

learning,

non-judgmental.

It will enrich your life.

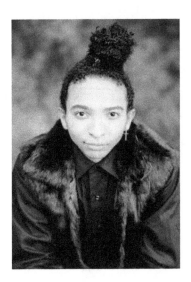

Be mindful, no two are alike no matter the DNA.

Each child requires original thinking and they have their own destiny.

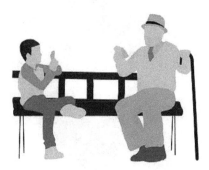

The elder need to be around the youth for energy and the current vantage.

The youth need to be around the elder to instill, inspire and teach to aspire.

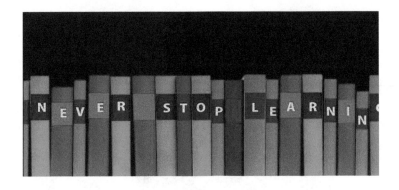

A teachable spirit is paramount.

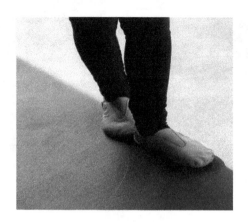

If you love discipline, you love knowledge.

Thoughts to note ...

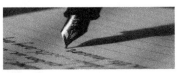

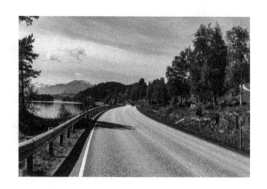

Know the guard rails for your life.

Stay pledged.

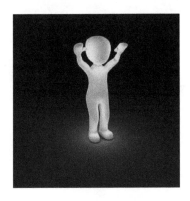

Too often you may believe or are told directly or subliminally, via friends, media, culture, scholars and the like that you should do, be, say, want, or react to life in ways that don't align with who YOU are or what you want.

When one is in the fullness of self, you will then truly be ready to share yourself fully with everyone and everything you encounter.

You will become light.

NOTE* Fullness of self will come in and out over periods of time. It will become permanent when you realize who you are, why you are breathing and what your purpose is.

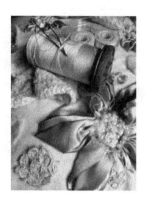

When life test the very stitching of your fabric, immediately - do not think, do whatever that thing is you do to reignite your spirit (body, mind and soul).

Run, read, pray, cook, coffee, yoga, knit, travel, play ball.

Busy the mind,

Busy the body,

Change the story.

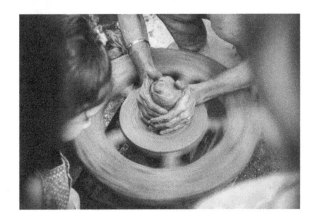

Failure is a judgement of an event. Failures shape you and can grow you if you are willing to let them.

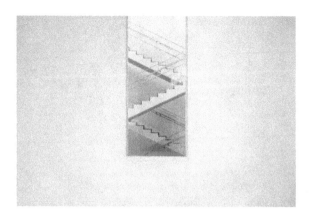

Let challenge make you better, not bitter. Re-frame your challenges.

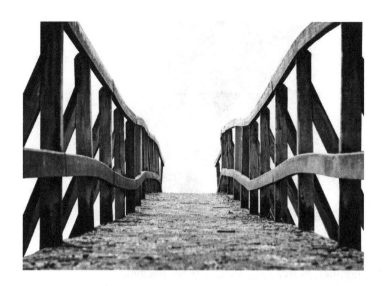

Transitional times provide new opportunities.

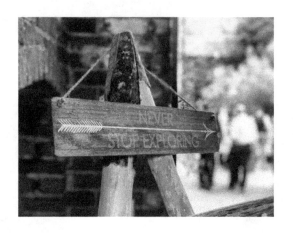

Remember, FORWARD PROGRESS always.

No Excuses!

NO EXCUSES!!

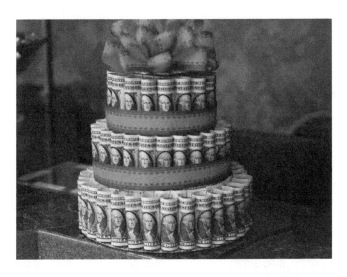

Find something you are good at and then do it everyday!

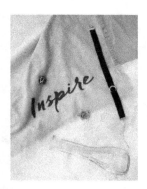

Words have great power.

Use **words** that stimulate, vivify and have positive purpose to all who hear them.

With actions aligned.

Thoughts to note ...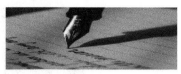

_____

_____

_____

_____

_____

_____

_____

_____

_____

_____

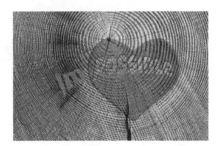

There will be many endless joyless days if you allow others have you believe any of the following;

◆ *you are what and who others say you are,*

◆ *you morph into what others say you need to be "more like" so you "fit in",*

◆ *you give up on your dreams because others communicate, in word, action or inaction, that you can not accomplish them.*

Emotional contagion is real. Choose company wisely.

Who you will ultimately become is quite possibly not who you, nor others believed is possible.

It is possible! YOU must BELIEVE in order for it to materialize.

Rise, go forward, do the work and meet your destiny with great impetus. Believe in who YOU say you are!

Each of us is born for a great purpose to a great destiny. Your beating heart is attestation.

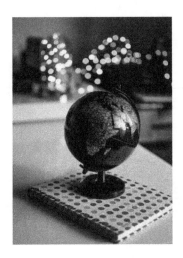

Education has a direct link to success. However, YOU acquire it …

discovery,

friendships,

personal reading,

travel,

university,

… find the piece of education that allows you to succeed.

Then give back to those around you and at large.

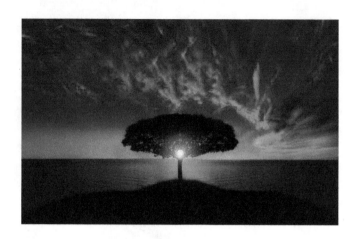

Knowledge comes.

Wisdom lingers.

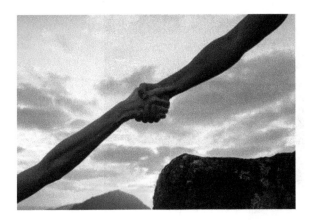

Reach forward towards success.

Reach back to help as many as you can with sensible, introspective initiative.

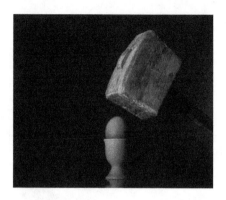

We are VULNERABLE, after success.

We are excited, tired from the work, celebrating the journey and accomplishment, away from our normal routine and environment where we think no one knows us or is watching closely.

It is good to pay attention to our decision-making markers at these times.

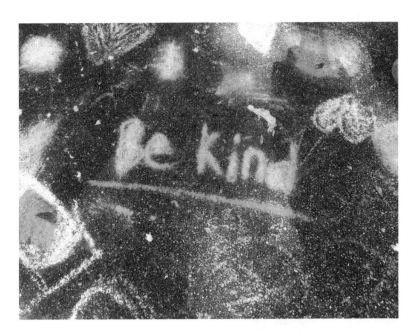

Be impressed by SINCERE,

true,

unplanned,

no expectation

KINDNESS.

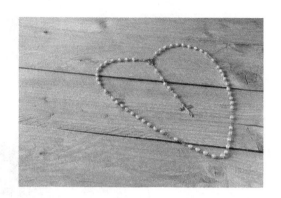

Value identity.

Know your Value.

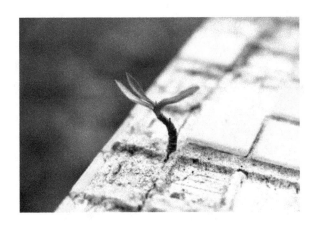

Believe in expectation.

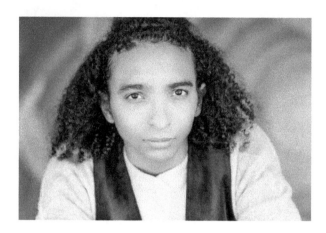

Every circumstance in life happens at the correct timing, for a purpose.

Thoughts to note ...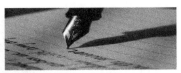

_____

_____

_____

_____

_____

_____

_____

_____

_____

_____

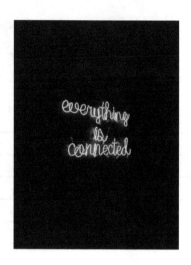

Establish connection and compatibility.

A favorite quote for growth seekers.

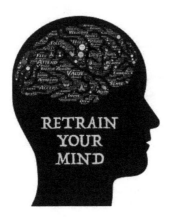

"You can't solve a problem with the same mind that created it", Einstein.

Learn something new everyday.

You were designed to succeed so that you can **help others**. The cycle repeats and this aids the advancement of all mankind.

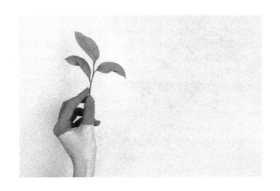

Growth and change are necessary for a JOY life.

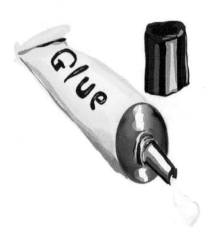

He who neglects discipline; despises himself.

Discipline is the glue that cements and is of supreme importance for any type of success.

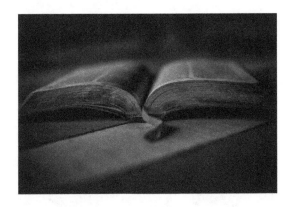

It is smart to dwell among the wise.

Wisdom is the beginning of knowledge and a sure way to honor, peace, and prosperity.

Friendship is powerful. It is Family.

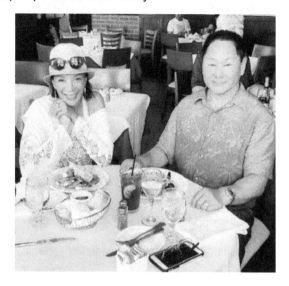

The most important ingredient in ANY relationship, is **FRIENDSHIP**.

True Friendship deserves a capital **F**.

Friendship lifts YOU up, supports YOU and is for YOU –

every time and always!

You can feel it.

If it does not lift you and you can not feel it - something to ponder.

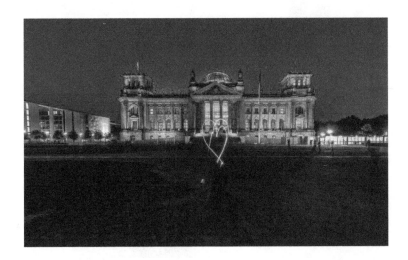

A big house is really nice.

A big "genuine" kind, loving heart is really necessary.

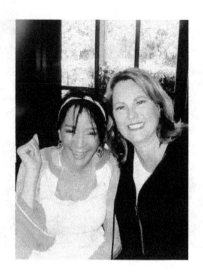

Friendship includes the freedom of truth.

Thoughts to note ...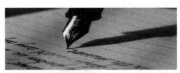

_____

_____

_____

_____

_____

_____

_____

_____

_____

_____

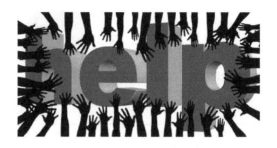

1. Give more and often.

2. Listen first and last.

3. Help others and allow them to help you.

No time, can't relate, not your turn, missed your turn, you always get the short stick?

Its OK. In the right timing, the first 3 rules will always lead to a propitious outcome.

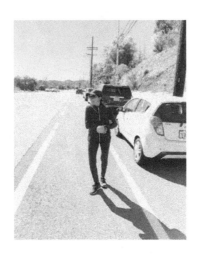

Aging healthy and gracefully involves movement - mind and body - everyday!

EVERYDAY.

NO EXCUSES.

Get moving - right now!

FRIENDS

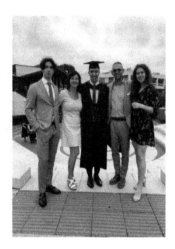

Support them
Show up for them.
Don't ask for the unnecessary.
Go to their shows.
Promote their good ideas.
Kindly let them know the shoes are wrong or the tie is off color.
Offer sincere congratulations when they achieve success.
Listen when they speak.
Help them when you can if necessary - <u>even when they don't ask</u>.
Listen to their life by listening to their stories.
Be the first to purchase their goods, services or products.
Be their shoulder or ear during timeouts and turbulence.
Be **genuinely** happy for them.
You will be a better FRIEND and it will bring YOU immense JOY.

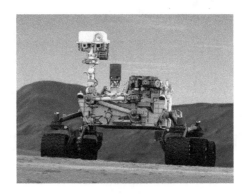

Curiosity is the key to longevity - and the true fountain of youth.

Keep reaching.

Keep learning.

Keep growing.

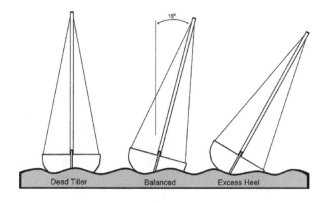

| Dead Tiller | Balanced | Excess Heel |

Pain is instructional. Be thankful for it - YOU are growing.

All pain comes with reason, even if it is unkind, unthinkable, unknowing.

The lesson starts at the occurrence of a painful situation, then proceeds to a midway marker. The goal is to arrive at the end marker, wiser and healed - where JOY awaits and you are now prepared to help others.

To beat pain - you must go through it (the lesson).

To get through it - you must have faith, be honest with yourself, the situation, and be willing to do (the work).

A winning outcome cannot come and remain without the WORK.

Our works are inescapable in every aspect of life.

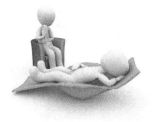

Identify emotions that tie you to the past.

LET GO of anyone and anything that does not move you forward, EVERY DAY.

Today is the day.

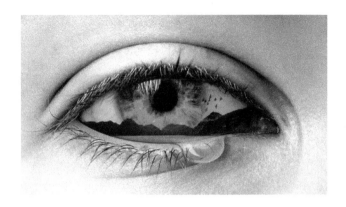

Have you ever seen selfless, helpful, genuine, want nothing, unconditional, no expectation assistance kind of LOVE?

It provokes tears and warming in the soul. This is LOVE.

This is beauty and beautiful.

Seek it. Be it.

It is absolutely wordless.

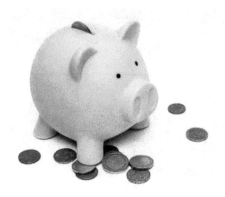

Invest in the worthwhile and the well-made, in everything.

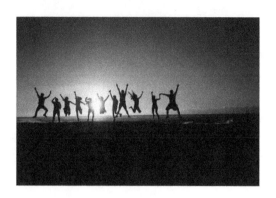

LIVE.

Everyday!

Visit a store you've never shopped, call an old friend from grade school - that was not a friend, prepare a new dish and share it with someone new and unexpecting, vacation and stay in a hotel in the city you reside, read to the elderly, visit a shelter, put on cologne, lipstick or a piece of fine jewelry and retire for the evening, learn a new language, tackle a new sport that challenges your mind, body and wallet.

LIVE.

Everyday.

Thoughts to note …

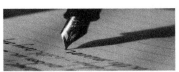

_____

_____

_____

_____

_____

_____

_____

_____

_____

_____

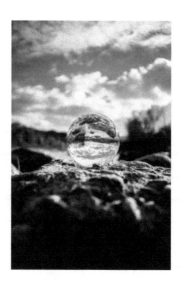

It is OK to be uncomfortable at times.

It presents growth opportunity and a chance to view life circum-stances through a different lens.

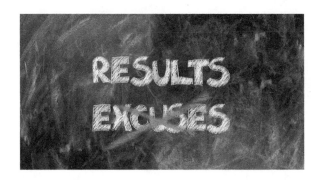

Make all the mistakes ~~excuses~~ you need to - but make NO excuses.

Mistakes become successes and are the results of trials turned TRIUMPHANT.

YOU can do it!

You must make a choice - ~~excuses~~ or do you want more JOY in life?

It's your choice - choose wisely.

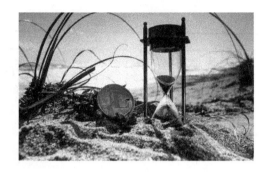

Timing matters.

Every circumstance in life happens at the correct timing, for a purpose.

The circumstance is the assignment.

If attention is paid, you learn the lesson inceptively, and move to the next episode.

The cycle repeats -

A - is continuous Joy in your journey.

F - is having to repeat assignment(s) many times.

Seek the A with exigency.

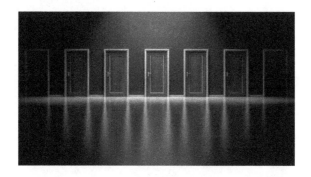

The more doors you open the more places you will go.

Some doors will require more mental fortitude and others more physical endurance.

Be tenacious.

YOU can do it!

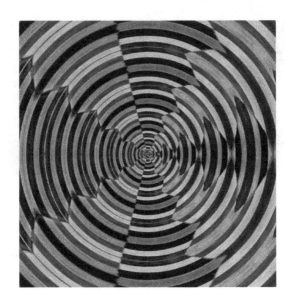

Be willing to go internal and explore your inner workings.

Your external will increase.

Inward work, strikes outward positive.

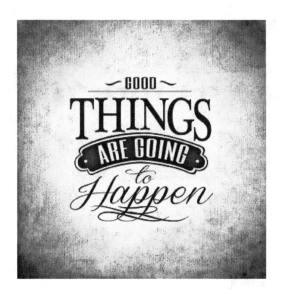

Rehearse good behavior daily.

It will lead to a lifetime of success.

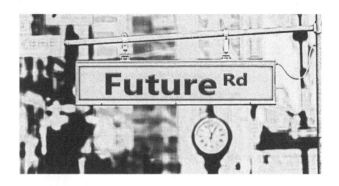

Are you defined by thoughts of the past?

Don't be - not even the mishaps of 30 minutes ago, yesterday or last year. Leave it.

Take the lesson - change the story.

The future is right now - in THIS moment.

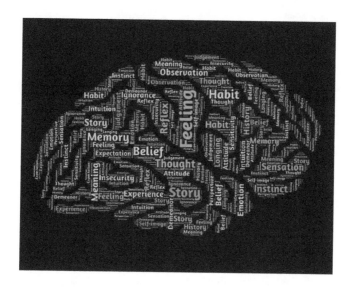

Think about, what you think about.

STOP! Right now - and really THINK about what you think about. This is pivotal. It is why YOU are where you are in your life.

90% of your thoughts are repetitive thoughts.

It is paramount they are prudent, progressive thoughts.

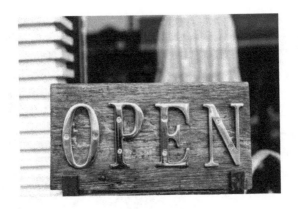

End thoughts are a thought language,

that breeds feeling thoughts, that contribute to the language of your body, your actions and ultimately your life.

Make POSITIVE thoughts your anchor.

Keep an open positive mindset.

Thoughts to note ...

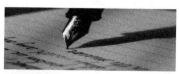

_____

_____

_____

_____

_____

_____

_____

_____

_____

_____

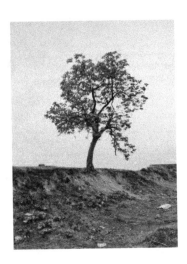

It's easier to lean in when you have faith, hope and peace of mind.

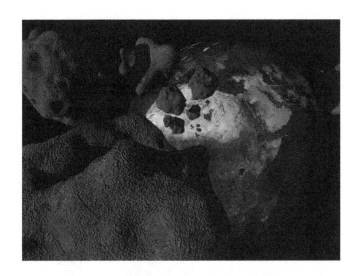

Moment of impact is change.

Change your mind, change your actions, change your life.

Game on!

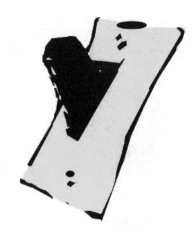

Old self to new self can happen in the flip of a switch.

Flip the switch.

Exercise your power.

Live the life you IMAGINE and more important, the life you are destined.

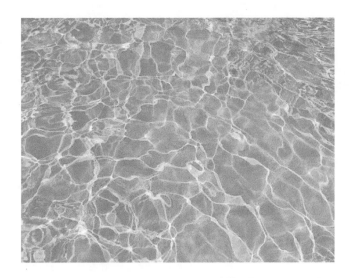

Whatever refreshes you on the way to your goals is a true, honest pleasure.

Identify what refreshes you – then be it and do it!

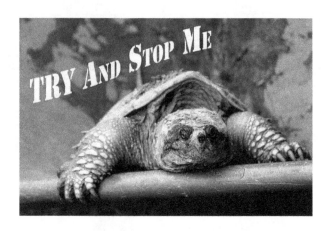

NEVER

GIVE

UP!

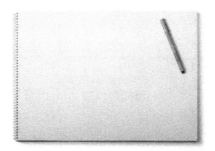

Have you ever written down on paper what the mission statement is for your life?

Do you know what the mission statement is for your life?

Are you living the mission statement of your life?

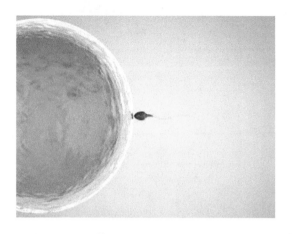

Are you living the life you were conceived to live?

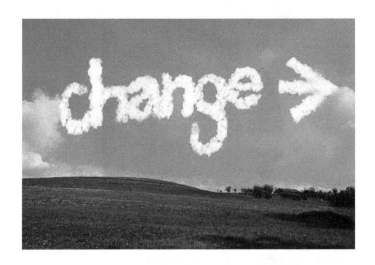

No conversion, without conviction.

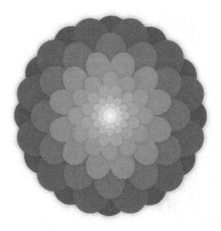

Love is the circulatory system of the body.

It doesn't matter if you don't speak Chinese, understand Hebrew in the written word, haven't traveled internationally, were not an A student, or don't know if first base is a reference to the game of football, soccer or baseball.

It is more important that you understand LOVE.

Thoughts to note ...

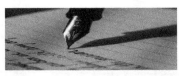

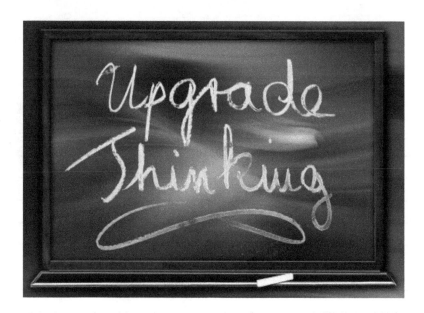

Learning

Becoming

Changing

MINDFULNESS -

When you get to the end of SELF, this is the beginning of knowing thy self.

To know where you are going, you must know YOU.

Then answers come and you learn your purpose.

STOP.

LISTEN.

THINK.

PROCEED, consciously.

(repeat often)

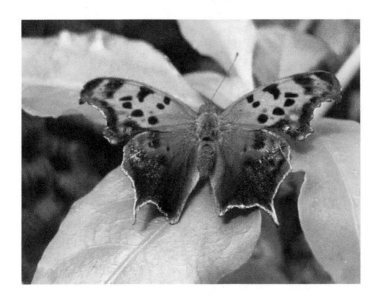

What would happen if we conformed to something higher, rather than conforming to whatever the current culture is?

Metamorphasis.

OVER POWERS

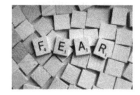

and

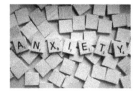

Fear and anxiety paralyzes faith.

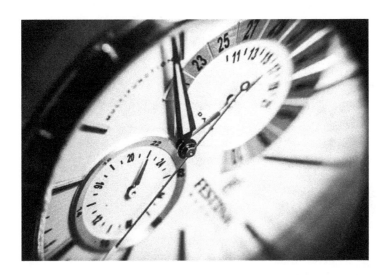

Do not disrespect time.

Do not leave it for later or tomorrow if it can be done NOW.

Do not wait until you have ALL the answers. You never will.

Opportunity is untimed and swift.

The unknown is the gift and it lends itself to possibility.

Be assiduous.

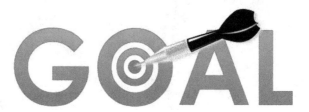

You can achieve most everything you want - just not all at once and certainly not without works.

Set your goals and get to work.

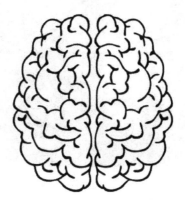

Be decisive. Do not vacillate in double mindedness.

It will cause your loyalties and your works to self and others to be divided, unstable and unsuccessful.

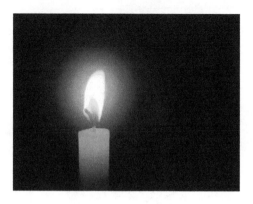

Character is formed in silence and darkness - when no one else is watching.

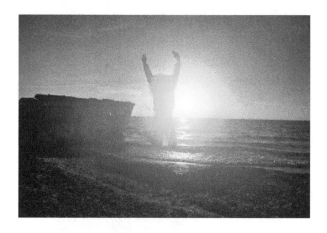

You are free when you are confidant in who you are, no matter where you are and no matter who you are with.

And, who you are NOT with.

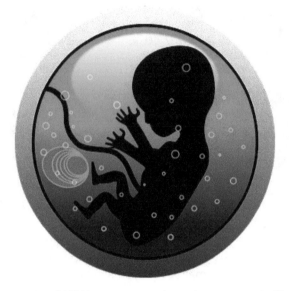

It does not matter HOW you came to be, what your early life circum-
stances may have been, or WHERE you are at the moment.

What matters is;

YOU are here now.

WHAT will you decide to DO and WHO will you decide to BE?

Answer the call that came with the gift of your beating heart.

YOU matter!

RISE!

Thoughts to note …

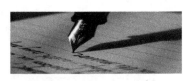

_____

_____

_____

_____

_____

_____

_____

_____

_____

_____

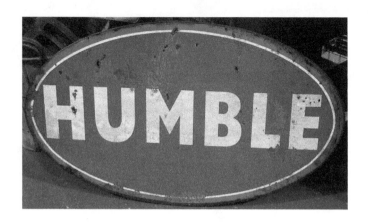

In order to be great -

you must be SINCERELY humble.

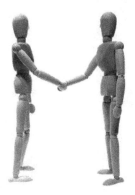

There will be and should be times in life when your growth game reaches new levels of maturation.

In these times, you will need to re-introduce yourself, to those who knew you a month prior, a year prior or 20 years prior.

Your growth game should always be in play and breaking new ground with regularity.

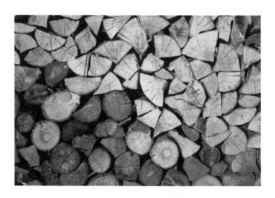

Overnight success is many years of hard work, determination and redefining what was once thought from youth, skill set and strategic planning.

Get to work.

The hill becomes lighter with diligence, maturity and perseverance.

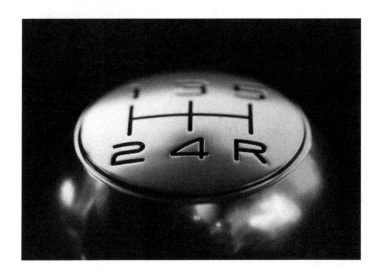

There comes a necessary time to let go of some people, places and/or things we liked, loved, or just held on to out of comfort, fear or lack of knowing how to transition and what the new transformation may present.

All relationships run a course, change and shift.

Personal soaring cannot continue with baggage that has satisfied its course - even well-liked baggage.

Important to pay keen attention to shifts and align accordingly.

Every relation has a direct effect on your JOY in life.

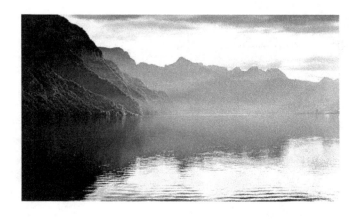

Every day - read and spend some time in silence.

It will come.

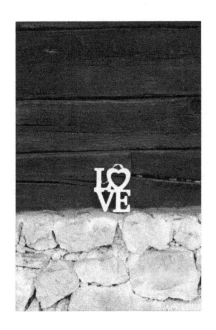

BEGIN and END with LOVE.

What is *GREATNESS*?

Ask a friend - do you want to achieve greatness in your life? The natural answer - probably a resounding YES! The conundrum; we turn inward, cogitating, how do I do that? How do I know when I have achieved this "greatness". What is the definition of greatness?

Books and scholars define greatness as: *The ability to achieve excellence in a specific area with masterful skill.* A concept of a state of superiority affecting a person or object in a particular place or area. Greatness can also be attributed to individuals who possess a natural ability to be better than all others.

Dictionary definition:

- "Unusual or considerable in degree, power or intensity."

- "Wonderful; first-rate; very good."

- "Notable; remarkable; exceptionally good."

Culturally defined, pursuing greatness resembles the following: Individuals motivated by self-interest, self-indulgence, and a false sense of self-sufficiency to pursue selfish ambition for the purpose of self-glorification.

So the real questions becomes: What is greatness and what does it mean to be **great - for YOU**?

It appears greatness in our modern world is tied to and defined by societal materialism and accomplishment. If you have money, status, collegiate education and power in position (and sometimes a false sense of it), then the world deems you great.

Is this REALLY greatness or what your greatness life looks like ?

Contrast those definition/s with perhaps greatness also being defined as; **helping others. This automatically makes YOU great.**

While there is no shame in money or material; Greatness and mastery cannot be defined by money and material. Your greatness is not tied to values society, culture, family or friends advise and foist upon you. That greatness usually does not come with the long term sustained feeling of satisfaction, and can be evanescent.

Greatness does not live in the house on the hill, own an island or have a certain title before or after it's name. Greatness takes time - to have it and recognize it. You may know a person or many of true greatness, that no one has ever heard of. Greatness does not always have a famous, well-known name or face.

Success can be happenstance, born of hard work, wealth or gifted, etc. It is not the desires of materialism in the pursuit of greatness that's bad, moreso the perceived definition; perhaps.

Greatness is serving others, which brings the server immense joy and how your greatness (material and otherwise) flows and grows.

In a word, true greatness is about **humility**. Genuine, **true** humility.

In a nutshell, if you are thinking about others and helping others along your journey, you will automatically achieve greatness personified.

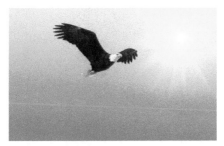

RISE, you matter

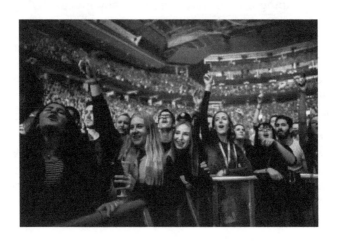

Show up with great temerity.

Knock 'em alive today - and every day!

Thoughts to note ...

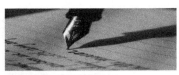

_____

_____

_____

_____

_____

_____

_____

_____

_____

_____

_____

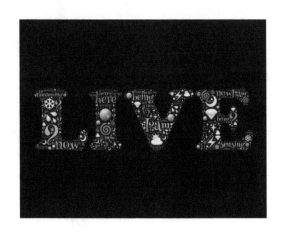

If it does not lift you up,

move you forward,

make you smile,

help you grow,

enrich your life,

educate you,

produce a great experience

or give you JOY on some level -

LET IT GO -

Right now!

A most important role.

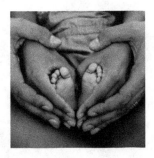

A parents role: love, teach and protect.

In youth, seek the child's interest, recognize their talent and help guide them relentlessly and selflessly to the pursuit of their interest and talent to the best ability. The goal is a wholly functioning and successful adult that is not just content in the world - but knows and has their purpose identified. This leads to their true JOY.

Ultimately, infants grow to adolescents, then to young adults and the time comes for them to navigate their own course.

Each adult has choices to make that will decide their course.

No matter the story of youth, the midpoint mania or the current path - right now, grow your knowledge, do the work, let love lead and choose JOY every single day!

Adulthood comes with the responsibility of owning YOUR destiny.

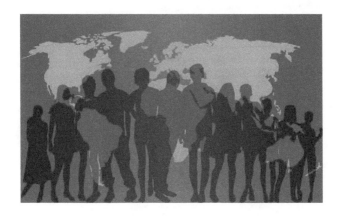

What if – all over the world, in every family, within every house-hold, each individual worked together genuinely, humbly, lovingly and collectively - no matter how challenging - to truly support each other, so that not only one in a generation would rise, but many?

It will take noble humility and produce planetary transmogrification.

GREATER THAN

How is it that a black or brown cow eats green grass, and produces white milk?

Sometimes we believe things that we can see, but cannot explain; then there are times we believe things that we cannot see or explain.

The only explanation .... there has to be something greater.

BELIEVE.

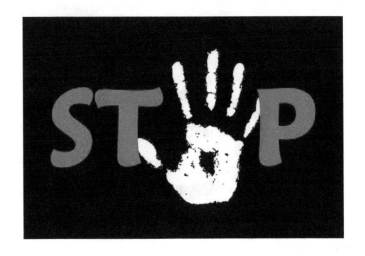

ANY ACTION

ANY ONE

ANY THING

ANY THOUGHT

and ANY LANGUAGE

That is not and does not foster enhancement and advancement.

RISE.

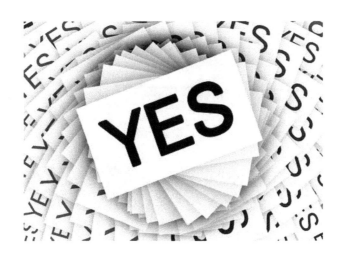

You can.

You will.

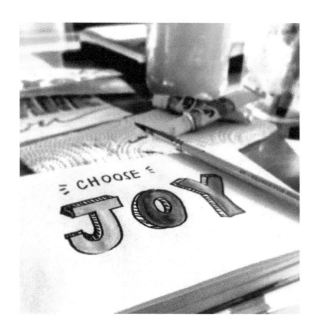

It is better to have JOY, than to always be right in dispute.

Keys to Joy

Love I Joy I Peace I Forbearance I Kindness I Goodness Faithfulness I Gentleness I Self-control.

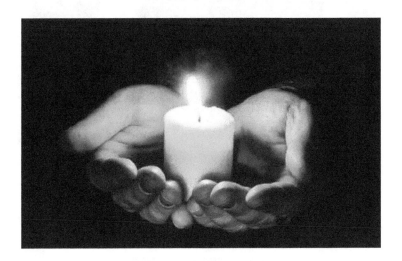

One can alter many.

Reach for the unreachable. Even if no one has done it before - someone has to be the first - why not YOU.

Do not allow old laid paths to hinder the unveiling of new paths, yet to be laid. Be a pioneer - it will positively affect you, your network, those associated with your networks and their networks.

Transfiguration.

RISE.

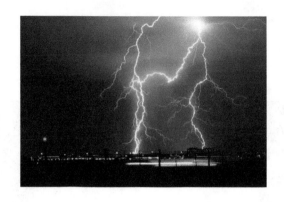

Dance

Laugh

Sing

….. like someone IS watching.

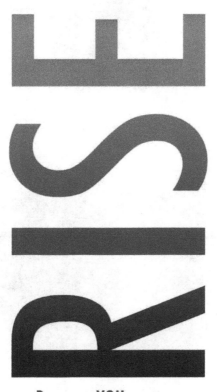

Because YOU matter.

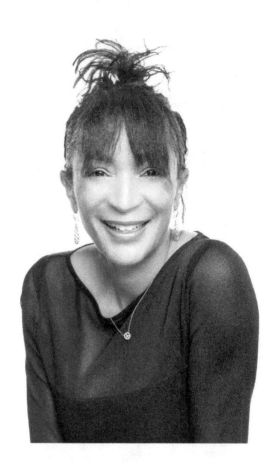

I am imperfectly rising every day -

striving towards amelioration.

RISE, you matter
141

CPSIA information can be obtained
at www.ICGtesting.com
Printed in the USA
JSHW040816060721
16543JS00001B/1